The Great Mediterra
Soups

By Jessica Petras

Your Free Gift- Get MORE out of your Diet!

As a way of saying thanks for your purchase, I'm offering a free mini-book that's exclusive to my book readers. Sticking to your diet or weight loss goals can be tough if you're walking around hungry all day. That's why I put together a set of quick tasty snack recipes made of ingredients you already have in your pantry to help you stay on track.

In **10 Quick & Easy Mediterranean Snacks that take 5 mins or less** I give you recipes for classic dishes like Fresh Zesty Bruschetta, Extra Creamy Hummus, and Spiced Nuts, to name a few, that are full of flavor and super easy to make. And in it you'll discover just how easy maintaining the Mediterranean Diet can be. You can download this free gift by going to: https://bit.ly/FreeMiniBook

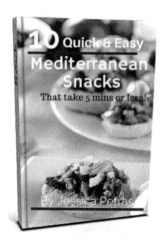

Introduction

By now you've probably heard about the most deliciously popular way of eating healthy and loving it, the Mediterranean Diet. What is the Mediterranean Diet? Simply put, the Mediterranean Diet is a scientifically researched plan for healthy eating that is abundant in flavor and nutrition. From the beautiful coasts of the Mediterranean to your table, these fabulous recipes are sure to please even the most discerning palate. Based upon ancient practices, which include using only the freshest of herbs, spices and ingredients, this wholesome plan allows you to take pleasure in what you consume, with complete confidence that you are doing the absolute best for your body. So many of the aches, pains and discomforts that we feel on a daily basis relate to what we consume day after day. Diets, which include processed sugars and flours as well as chemicals and preservatives can promote fatigue, chronic pain and many other uncomfortable and potentially dangerous afflictions. Feeling better can be as simple as changing the way we eat. The Mediterranean Diet offers a delicious alternative that will treat your body the way that it deserves to be treated – you'll feel the difference!

Save Time and Feel Great!

One of the challenges that we face in trying to live a healthy lifestyle, which includes fresh, wholesome foods, is finding adequate time for meal preparation. Part of the secret to success in following a healthy eating program is having a tasty and extensive collection of recipes that require minimal time and effort to prepare. As you explore this delightful collection of our most favorite Mediterranean soups and salads, you'll begin to realize just how easy it is to prepare and serve gourmet-quality foods that are power-packed with all of the nutrients that you'll need to lose weight, increase your energy level and feel healthy and strong. Delicious, nutritious and satisfying, these amazing recipes will give you the boost that you need to effectively maintain your healthy new Mediterranean Diet.

Salads

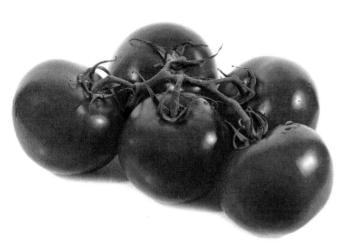

Tomato Mozzarella and Olive Penne Salad

Savory and satisfying, you'll love this decadent-tasting dish of pasta perfection.

Ingredients:

- 2 large tomatoes, cut into wedges
- 1 medium onion, thinly sliced
- 3/4 cup Italian salad dressing, divided
- 1/2 cup slivered fresh basil leaves or 1 tablespoon dried basil leaves
- 1/2 cup sliced pitted ripe olives
- 1 (12 ounce) package of Penne, uncooked
- 1/2 pound cubed mozzarella cheese

Instructions:

Get a large bowl and stir in the onion, tomatoes, basil, olives and ½ cup salad dressing. Set aside. Prepare and cook the pasta based on the directions written on its package. For faster cooling, rinse the pasta using cold water.

Get another large bowl and toss in the marinated veggies prepared earlier. Add the cooled pasta, mozzarella cheese and left over salad dressing. Cover the bowl and put it in the fridge. Best served cold.

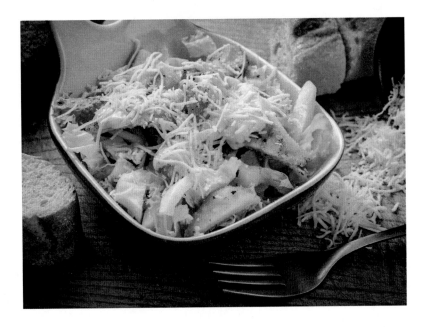

Caesar Salad

Tangy, crunchy and just a bit salty, this restaurant favorite is a delicious quick-fix.

Ingredients:

- 2 small garlic cloves, minced
- 1 teaspoon anchovy paste

- 2 tablespoons freshly squeezed lemon juice, from one lemon
- 1 teaspoon Dijon mustard
- 1 teaspoon Worcestershire sauce
- 1 cup mayonnaise
- 1/2 cup freshly grated Parmigiano-Reggiano
- 1/4 teaspoon salt
- 1/4 teaspoon freshly ground black pepper
- 2 heads **romaine lettuce** (rinsed, patted dry, wilted outer leaves discarded)

Instructions:

Get a medium sized bowl. Add in the anchovy paste, lemon juice, Worcestershire sauce, Dijon mustard and garlic. Add the remaining ingredients which namely salt, pepper, mayonnaise and Parmigiano-Reggiano. Whisk until everything is well combined. Give it a taste and adjust according to your preference. Rinse lettuce clean and cut into 1 ½ inch chunks. Place cut lettuce into a large bowl, drizzle with dressing. Enjoy!

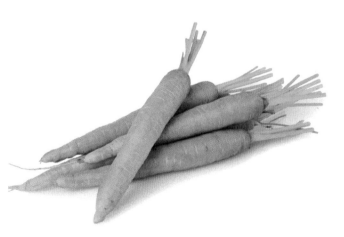

Crispy Carrot Salad with Plump Golden Raisins

Filled with sweet substance, this colorful treat is sure to please!

Ingredients:

- 1 pound large sweet carrots, peeled
- 3 tablespoons golden raisins
- 2/3 cup mint leaves, cut into chiffonade or 1/4-inch julienne
- 2 teaspoons freshly squeezed lemon juice
- 1 tablespoon extra-virgin olive oil
- Salt and freshly ground black pepper

Instructions:

Use the grater blade from a food processor or a box grater and grate the carrots. Get a medium sized bowl. Combine the lemon juice, olive oil, golden raisins and mint. Add salt and pepper to taste. Toss all the ingredients. Serve and enjoy.

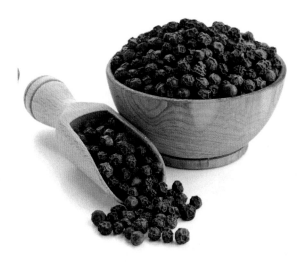

Spicy Pepper & Tomato Cucumber Salad

Refreshing with just a bit of kick, this delightful dish will tempt your taste buds.

Ingredients:

- 2 large tomatoes (or 4 medium), chopped
- 1/2 large cucumber, peeled and diced
- 1/2 yellow pepper, seeded and chopped
- 1 small onion, diced
- 2 cloves garlic, minced
- 1/2 cup parsley, finely chopped
- 2 tablespoons lemon juice
- 1 tablespoon red wine vinegar
- 2 tablespoons Spicy V-8 (or tomato juice)
- generous grating black pepper
- 1/2 teaspoon paprika
- 1/4 teaspoon cumin
- salt to taste (optional)

Instructions:

Mix all the ingredients in a bowl. You can serve it immediately after preparation or you can chill it for an hour before serving. This is perfect when paired with pita and hummus. Or you can also top it over a green salad.

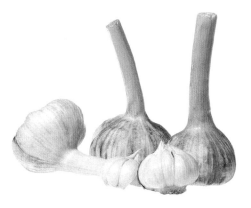

Garlic Chicken White Bean Salad

Hearty and delicious, this fiber and protein-packed selection is the new definition of comfort food.

Ingredients:

For the Salad:

- 2 cups coarsely chopped skinless, boneless rotisserie chicken
- 1 cup chopped tomato
- 1/2 cup thinly sliced red onion
- 1/3 cup sliced fresh basil
- 2 (16-ounce) cans cannellini beans or other white beans, rinsed and drained

For the Dressing:

- 1/4 cup red wine vinegar
- 2 tablespoons extra virgin olive oil
- 1 tablespoon fresh lemon juice
- 2 teaspoons Dijon mustard
- 1/2 teaspoon salt
- 1/4 teaspoon freshly ground black pepper
- 2 garlic cloves, minced

Instructions:

Salad Preparation: Add in the first five ingredients in a large mixing bowl. Combine all the ingredients by stirring it gently. Set aside.

Dressing Preparation: Get another bowl. Whisk the vinegar along with the remaining ingredients. Pour it over your prepared salad and toss carefully. Serve and enjoy this sumptuous treat.

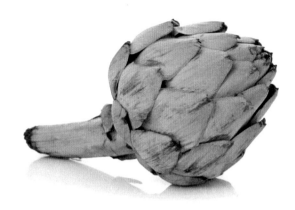

Couscous Salad with Artichokes and Tomatoes

This textural delight features savory tidbits to tempt the palate.

Ingredients:
- 1 (16 oz.) package couscous (we used World Market's Tri-Color Couscous)
- 2 cups halved grape tomatoes
- 2 cups jarred artichoke hearts, drained and chopped
- 1 1/2 cups chopped kalamata olives, pits removed
- 1/2 cup chopped fresh basil
- For the dressing:
- 1/2 cup olive oil
- Juice of 2 large lemons
- 3 cloves garlic, minced
- 2 teaspoons chopped fresh oregano
- 1 tablespoon chopped fresh basil
- Salt and pepper, to taste

Instructions:

Prepare the couscous. Make sure to follow the directions written in the package. Get a large bowl. Place couscous in the large bowl. Use a fork to fluff it. Add in basil, kalamata olives, tomatoes and artichoke hearts. Set aside.

Whisk lemon juice, garlic, basil, oregano and olive oil in a small mixing bowl. Add the dressing over the prepared couscous and mix well by stirring. If you want, you can adjust the taste accordingly by adding salt and pepper. Serve and enjoy.

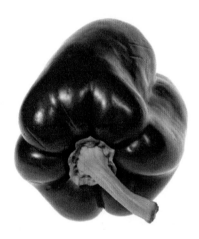

Chopped Chicken Salad with Olives Red Pepper and Feta

You'll be the envy of everyone in the lunch room with this colorful and tasty dish.

For the Dressing:
- 1/4 cup red wine vinegar
- 2 T Balsamic Vinegar
- 1 T Dijon Mustard

- 1 tsp. Italian Seasoning herb blend
- 1/2 tsp. Vege-Sal or salt
- Fresh ground black pepper to taste, about 1/2 tsp.
- 1 Cup extra virgin olive oil

For each salad:
- 1 cup diced leftover chicken breast, cut into pieces 1/2 inch square
- 1/4 cup chopped red pepper, cut into pieces 1/2 inch square
- 1/4 cup black olives, cut in half
- 2 large handfuls chopped romaine lettuce
- 2 T crumbled Feta cheese

Instructions:
Prepare a measuring cup or a mixing bowl. Combine all of the ingredients except for the olive oil. Gradually add in the olive oil and whisk it up until all of the ingredients have been combined well.

Create the dressing and set it aside to allow the flavors to blend as you prepare the ingredients needed for your salad.

Slice chicken, olives and red bell pepper. Place these ingredients in a bowl. Toss it with 1 to 2 Tbsp. dressing and let it sit while you prepare the other ingredients.

Wash and chop lettuce in small, bite sized portions. Dry it using paper towels. Crush the feta cheese.

Get a salad bowl and put in the chopped lettuce. You can also adjust the taste by adding more dressing. Top the lettuce with the marinated chicken, olives and red bell pepper. Sprinkle the top with the crumbled feta cheese. Serve and enjoy.

You can keep the remaining dressing in the fridge for a couple of weeks. Just make sure that you allow the dressing to come to room temp and shake it after every use. If in case you do not wish to prepare the dressing, you can use your desired bottled dressing as an alternative.

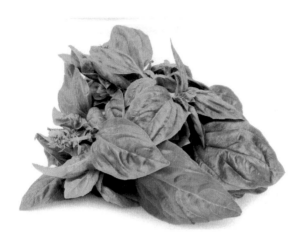

Insalata Caprese (Tomato, Mozzarella and Basil Salad)

Fresh basil and tomato sing in contrast to creamy mozzarella in this classic Mediterranean salad.

Ingredients:
- 4 large ripe tomatoes, sliced 1/4 inch thick
- 1 pound fresh mozzarella cheese, sliced 1/4 inch thick
- 1/3 cup fresh basil leaves
- 3 tablespoons extra virgin olive oil
- fine sea salt to taste
- freshly ground black pepper to taste

Instructions:
Prepare a large plate. Place the tomato slices first and then the mozzarella cheese and finally, the basil leaves. Make sure they overlap for better presentation. Drizzle the top with olive oil. Add salt and pepper to taste. Serve!

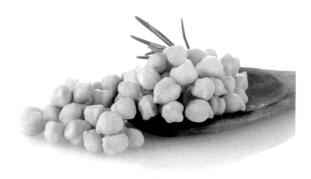

Arugula and Chickpea Salad with Sweet Peppers and Lemon Dressing

Not your ordinary salad, the flavor, texture and crunch of this tasty favorite will delight you.

Ingredients:
- 2 15 0z cans garbanzo beans, drained
- 1 Cup chopped roasted red pepper, drained
- 1/4 Cup extra virgin olive oil
- 1/2 fresh lemon squeezed
- 1/4 teaspoon kosher salt
- 1/4 teaspoon fresh cracked black pepper
- 1 bag of fresh arugula

Instructions:
Put in the pepper and the garbanzo beans in a bowl.

Add in the lemon juice, olive oil, pepper and salt to taste in a separate bowl. Whisk until well combined. Toss it over the prepared beans. Toss it again until evenly coated. Get a spoonful of arugula leaves and add it in. Toss it again.
You can serve it immediately after preparation or let it cool first on the fridge.

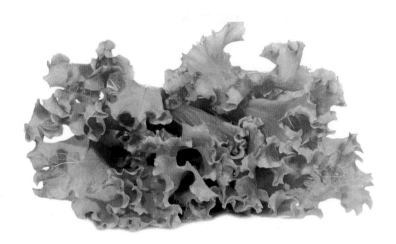

Light Tuna and Mixed Greens Antipasto Salad

Tangy and savory, this healthy and nutritious salad is sure to satisfy.

Ingredients:
- 1 15- to 19-ounce can beans, such as chickpeas, black-eyed peas or kidney beans, rinsed
- 2 5- to 6-ounce cans water-packed chunk light tuna, drained and flaked (see Note)
- 1 large red bell pepper, finely diced
- 1/2 cup finely chopped red onion
- 1/2 cup chopped fresh parsley, divided
- 4 teaspoons capers, rinsed
- 1 1/2 teaspoons finely chopped fresh rosemary
- 1/2 cup lemon juice, divided
- 4 tablespoons extra-virgin olive oil, divided
- Freshly ground pepper, to taste
- 1/4 teaspoon salt
- 8 cups mixed salad greens

Instructions:
Prepare a medium sized bowl. Put in the beans, bell pepper, tuna, capers, onion, parsley, lemon juice (1/4cup) and 2 tbsp. oil. Add pepper.
Get another large bowl and combine the remaining lemon juice (1/4 cup), salt and 2 tbsp. oil. Add in the salad greens and toss to coat evenly. Get 4 plates and divide the salad. Top each plate with your prepared tuna salad. Serve and enjoy.

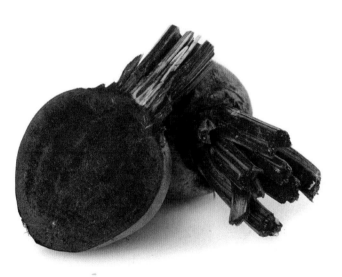

Beet Goat Cheese Arugula Salad with Lemon Mustard Drizzle

Deliciously different, the combination of flavors in this light yet hearty dish is not to be missed.

Salad Ingredients:
- Beets - (boiled until a fork easily goes in it, about an hour, or you can use canned beets), peeled, sliced into strips

- Fresh arugula - rinsed, patted dry with a paper towel
- Goat cheese - Chevre
- Walnuts - chopped

For the Dressing:
- Olive oil
- Lemon
- Dry powdered mustard
- Sugar
- Salt and pepper

Instructions:
For the salad dressing, combine lemon, powdered mustard, sugar, salt and pepper, and olive oil.

For the salad, prepare it according to the amount that you want to serve. Combine the arugula leaves, beet juliennes, crumbled goat cheese in a plate or bowl and garnish it with chopped walnuts. You can use the dressing described earlier or a vinaigrette dressing as an alternative.

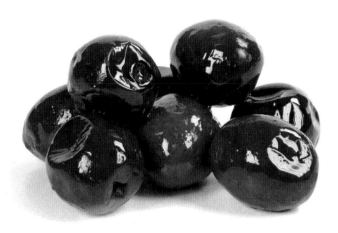

Classic Nicoise Salad

This healthy Nicoise is flavorfully naughty, but nutritionally nice.

Ingredients:
- 1 tablespoon Dijon mustard
- 1/4 cup extra virgin olive oil
- 1 tablespoon red wine vinegar
- 3 cups mixed greens, washed and dried
- 1/2 cup green beans, fresh, cooked
- 2 plum tomatoes, diced
- 1/2 cucumber seeded and chopped
- 1/2 small red onion, thinly sliced into rounds
- 1/2 cup black olives, pitted
- 1 cup boiled potatoes, sliced
- 1 can solid white Albacore tuna, drained
- 2 hard-boiled eggs, sliced into quarters
- 4 anchovy filets
- 2 tablespoons capers

Instructions:
Whisk the olive oil, vinegar and mustard in a bowl until smooth and then set aside.
Assemble the greens on a plate and add in the green beans, cucumbers, tomatoes, olives, potatoes and onions on the sides of the bowl. Top the greens with tuna.

Put in the anchovies and hard boiled eggs on the side and garnish the salad with capers. Put some mustard dressing on top of the salad. Serve and Enjoy.

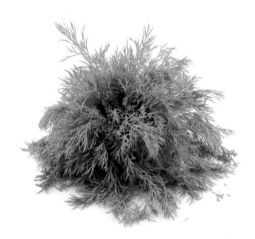

Fresh Dill and Feta Cucumber Salad

Light and refreshing, this Mediterranean salad-with-substance is sure to be a go-to favorite.

Ingredients:
- 1 English cucumber chopped or sliced
- 1/4 cup Greek yogurt
- 1/4 cup Feta cheese
- 1/4 cup chopped fresh dill
- salt and pepper to taste

Instructions:
Combine all the ingredients in a bowl. Serve and Enjoy.

Soups

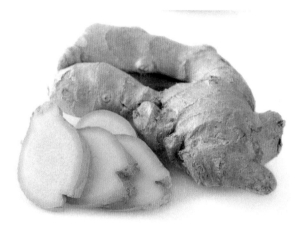

Ginger Lentil Soup with Balsamic and Cilantro

Fresh and fragrant, this healthy and hearty soup is sure to please.

Ingredients:
- 1 tablespoon canola oil
- 1 cup pre-chopped onion
- 1 tablespoon minced fresh garlic
- 1 tablespoon minced peeled fresh ginger
- 1 1/2 tablespoons curry powder
- 1/8 teaspoon ground red pepper
- 3 cups fat-free, lower-sodium chicken broth
- 1 1/2 tablespoons balsamic vinegar
- 2 (8-ounce) packages steamed lentils
- 2 cups fresh baby spinach
- 1/4 teaspoon kosher salt
- 1/4 teaspoon freshly ground black pepper

- 1/4 cup chopped fresh cilantro, divided
- 1/4 cup plain 2% reduced-fat Greek yogurt

Instructions:

Heat a medium sized skillet over medium fire or heat. Add some oil into the pan. Swirl the added oil in the pan to evenly coat. Put in the onions and sauté for about 3 minutes.

Add ginger and garlic and sauté for another minute. Add in the red bell pepper and curry powder. Cook for another 30 seconds while constantly stirring. Put in the broth, lentils and vinegar. Adjust the heat from medium to high until it boils. Lower the heat and let it simmer for another 5 minutes.

Halve the lentil mixture and put it in a blender. Take out the center portion of the blender cover, to reveal the opening. Get a clean towel and position it on the opening portion of the blender cover. Blend the mixture until it becomes smooth. Add salt, pepper and the blended mixture onto the pan. Constantly stir it until the spinach wilts. Add in 2 tbsp. cilantro.

Best served with remaining cilantro and yogurt.

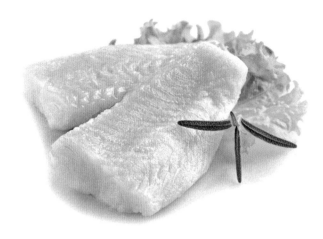

Hearty Italian Fish Soup

Filled with flavor this bold offering will warm you from the inside out.

Ingredients:
- 2 tablespoons olive oil
- 1 large sweet onion, chopped (about 2 cups)
- 1/4 cup dry white wine or Chicken Broth
- 4 cups Vegetable Broth or Chicken Broth
- 1 can (14.5 ounces) diced tomatoes, un-drained
- 24 (8 ounces) sliced fresh mussels, scrubbed and beards removed
- 1 pound firm white fish fillets (cod, haddock or halibut), cut into 1-inch pieces
- 1/2 pound fresh or thawed frozen large shrimp, peeled and deveined
- Shredded fresh basil leaves

Instructions:
Prepare a six quart pot. Heat the pot on medium heat. Put in the onion. Cook until it is soft.

Put in the wine and cook for another minute. Add in the tomatoes and stir in the broth. Heat it until it comes to a boil. Adjust the heat settings from medium to low. Add in the shrimps, fish and the mussels. Cover the pot and cook it until the mussels are open. The shrimps should be cooked thoroughly and the fish should easily flake with a fork. Any mussels that don't open should be discarded. Add salt and pepper to taste. Add in basil for garnish.

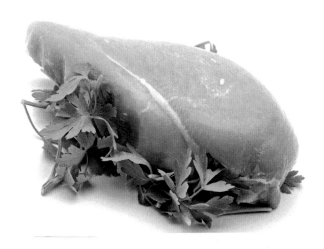

Greek Diced Chicken and Garbanzo Bean Soup

Packed with protein, you'll love this tasty dish.

Ingredients:
- 3-4 cups diced, cooked chicken
- 1 can (15.5 oz.) garbanzo beans (chickpeas)
- 1 onion, diced small

- 1 can (14.5 oz) petite diced tomatoes with juice
- 2 T finely chopped fresh oregano (or use 2-3 tsp. dried oregano)
- 1 tsp. minced garlic (or use garlic puree from a jar)
- 1 tsp. Greek Seasoning (If you don't have Greek Seasoning, see note below.)
- 1 tsp. vegetable soup base (I like Better than Bouillon Organic Vegetable Base)
- 6-8 cups chicken stock, homemade or canned
- 1/2 cup chopped fresh parsley
- crumbled Feta cheese for serving (optional, but very good)

Instructions:
Cut the chicken into portions until you come up with 3-4 cups. Rinse off garbanzo beans well in colander until foam disappears. Finely chop the oregano and onion. Get your crockpot. Place all the ingredients except for the parsley. Cover and cook it over medium heat for 8 to 10 hours.

Crumble the feta cheese and chop the parsley. Spoon over half of the chopped parsley and add it to the soup. Cook it for a couple of minutes more. Serve it hot and don't forget the extra chopped parsley and crushed feta.

Basically, Greek Seasoning is composed of black pepper, marjoram, lemon peel, oregano, garlic and salt. You can make use of a mixture of whatever you have if in case you don't have Greek seasoning available.

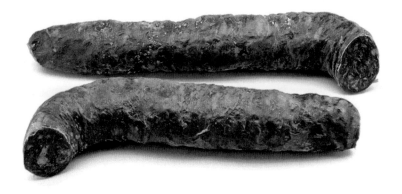

Quick White Bean & Chorizo Soup

Spicy and decadent, you'll thoroughly enjoy this magnificent Mediterranean soup.

Ingredients:
- 4 ounces chorizo sausage, chopped
- 1 small onion, chopped
- 2 cloves garlic, coarsely chopped
- 1 can (15 oz. to 19 oz.) cannellini or white kidney beans, rinsed and drained
- 5 cups water
- 2 Knorr ® Tomato Bouillon with Chicken flavor Cubes, crumbled
- 2 Tbsp. chopped fresh cilantro

Instructions:
Prepare a small saucepot. Brown the chorizo over medium-high heat while stirring every once and a while. Add in the onion and then cook for another 4 minutes and up until it is gold in color. Add in beans and garlic and stir it to evenly coat the beans for another 1 minute. Add Knorr Tomato Bouillon cubes with chicken flavor and water. Bring it to a boil. Lower the heat setting and then simmer it for about 15 minutes. Add in the cilantro. Serve and enjoy.

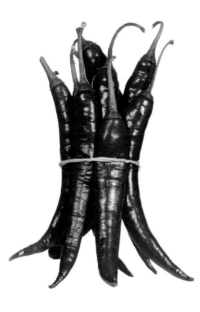

Mediterranean Spiced Tomato Soup w/ Chickpeas

A new twist on an old favorite, this Spiced Tomato Soup is meant to be sipped and savored.

Ingredients:
- 3 garlic cloves (minced)
- 3 red chili peppers
- 1/2 tsp red pepper flakes
- 1 tsp ground coriander
- 3/4 tsp coarse salt
- 1/8 tsp caraway seeds
- 2 tbsps extra-virgin olive oil
- 15 ozs garbanzo (drained and rinsed)
- 11/2 cups tomatoes with juice (crushed canned)
- 1/2 cup roasted red peppers (drained jarred, rinsed)

- 31/2 cups low sodium store bought chicken stock (or homemade)
- sour cream (for serving)
- parsley sprigs (for garnish)

Instructions:
Crush the garlic, salt, caraway, coriander and chilies using a mortar and pestle or as an alternative, the back of the spoon to create a paste.

Place a saucepan and heat the oil on medium-high heat. Put in the garlic blend and cook it for 3 minutes or until tender.
Stir in the red peppers (roasted), tomatoes, chickpeas and stock. Simmer it for another 15 minutes and stir it constantly. Let it cool for a few minutes.

Get your blender and puree the soup. Work it in batches. You can rewarm it if needed. Divide it among the prepared bowls. Top each bowl serving with sour cream and parsley.

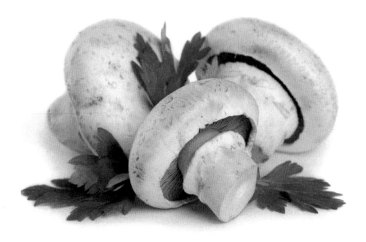

Classic Italian Vegetable Soup (Minestrone)

This is minestrone at its finest – healthy and tasty.

Ingredients:
- 1 lb lean ground Beef
- 4 ozs sliced mushrooms
- 1 yellow onion (diced)
- 4 cloves garlic (chopped)
- 2 stalks celery (sliced)
- 1 cup carrots (chopped)
- 141/2 ozs stewed tomatoes (or diced)
- 1 tbsp dried oregano
- 4 cups beef broth
- 2/3 cup elbow pasta (dried, to add later)
- kosher salt (add to taste at the table)

Instructions:

Prepare your slow cooker (6 quart). Take the first 4 ingredients on the list and brown it on your stovetop. Remove the fat by draining it. Put the meat in your slow cooker and add in the veggies. Add the beef broth, tomatoes and oregano. Stir it to combine well and cover the slow cooker. Cook it on low heat for 8 ½ hours. Add in the dry pasta and stir. Adjust the heat to high and cook for 30 minutes more or until pasta becomes tender.
Serve in bowls and topped with parmesan cheese.

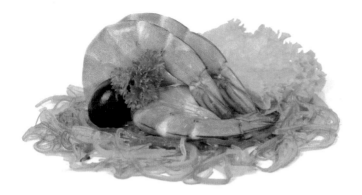

Cioppino with Sea Bass Shrimp and Clams

Savory seafood delights abound in this classic Mediterranean dish.

Ingredients:
- 3 lbs halibut (sea bass, or other firm white fish, cut into inch-long cubes)
- 2 lbs Dungeness crabs (or more cooked, hard shell)
- 1 lb large shrimp (or more of)
- 2 lbs littleneck clams (and/or mussels)
- 1/2 cup olive oil
- 11/2 cups chopped onion (1 large onion)
- 1 cup chopped bell pepper (1 large bell pepper)
- 3 cloves garlic (minced)
- 1 tsp salt
- 28 ozs tomatoes
- broth (from the mollusks)
- 2 cups red wine
- 2 cups tomato juice
- 2 cups fish (or shellfish stock)
- basil
- bouquet
- salt
- pepper
- 1/2 cup parsley (minced, for garnish)

Instructions:

Place the mussels and clams in a pot. Add in 2 cups of water. Steam it until the mollusks open up. Put aside. Drain the cooking broth and reserve it for later.

Separate the legs from the body of the crab. Open up the crab shell using a nutcracker so the meat could easily be taken out when it is served. Split the body in two and cut every half to another set of halves. You can choose to leave the meat inside the crab parts but that will mean much more work for the eater. You also have another option which is to remove the meat from the crab parts. When you pick the crab meat, always keep it in large portions. Retain the upper casing of the crab for creating stock.
Please note you can utilize well prepared shellfish or perhaps fish stock, or you could create your very own. If you're not creating your very own stock, you could dispose of the crab upper shell body. When well-prepared shellfish stock isn't readily available, I will mix a few well prepared fish stock along with clam juice.
Divide the shrimp shells on the backside and take away the black colored vein. The simplest way to get this done, without taking out the shell, would be to place the shrimp on the side and then stick in a little blade to the big end of the shrimp, along with the knife facing outward form its back (away from your hands and the shrimps). Once you've separated the shells of the shrimp, you could flip the knife in the direction of the shrimp, and slice in just a little to uncover the black vein. Take out the vein while you could. You could likely also utilize a set of kitchen scissors to slice the shrimp's backs.

On the other hand, you could shell and devein the shrimps. You will get more flavor with the shells on while it is going to be a lot easier to it with the shells off.
Using an 8 quart deep covered pot, sauté the bell peppers and onions over medium heat in olive oil right until it tender. Put in the garlic and sauté it again for another minute. Add the salt, pepper, tomato juice, stock, herb bouquet, mollusks broth, tomatoes and red wine. Cook and simmer without the cover for 20 minutes. Take out the herb bouquet. Adjust taste according to your preference.

Add in the fish and cover the pot. Cook it for about 3 to 5 minutes or up until the fish has been cooked well. Add in the steamed mollusks, shrimp and crabmeat. Heat it until the shrimps are cooked for another 3 to 5 minutes or up until the shrimps turn bright pink in color. Make sure that you do not overcook it.

Serve the soup in big bowls together with the shells. Top it off with minced parsley. Best served with Italian or French bread and a glass of wine. Make sure you prepare extra bowls for the shell, small forks and nut crackers for the crabs.

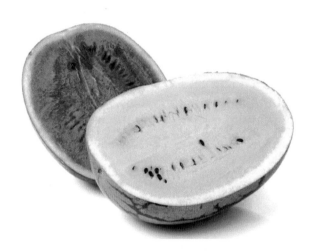

Watermelon Gazpacho with lime and Cilantro

Cool and refreshing, this unique Mediterranean interpretation of the traditional Spanish dish is sure to please.

Ingredients:
- 14 ozs diced tomatoes (drained)
- 1 cup watermelon (chopped and seeds removed, Red will do but try yellow if you can find it. It's much sweeter.)
- 1 can tomato juice

- 1/2 cup bloody Mary mix
- 1 tsp chopped parsley
- 2 tbsp fresh lime juice
- salt
- pepper
- lime
- cilantro

Instructions:
Prepare your food processor. Combine all of the listed ingredients and blend it well or until smooth. If you like chunky gazpacho, pulse the food processor to mix the ingredients to small chunks. Add salt and pepper to taste. Top it with lime wedges and cilantro.

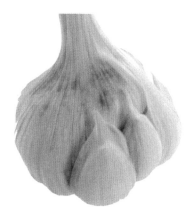

Super Simple Spicy Garlic Soup and Poached Eggs

This easy to fix dish is out of this world with flavor!

Ingredients:
- 1 head garlic cloves (peeled and thinly sliced)
- 3 tbsp olive oil

- 8 baguette (1/2-inch-thick, slices)
- 1 qt chicken stock (or broth)
- 1/2 tsp hot red pepper flakes (dried)
- 4 large eggs
- 1/2 cup cilantro sprigs (packed small fresh)
- 4 lime wedges

Instructions:
Prepare a 10 inch deep skillet and place it under low heat. Put in the oil and cook garlic while stirring often until it turns pale golden and tender for about 8-10 minutes. Use a spoon to transfer the cooked garlic in a bowl. Add in the slices of bread on to the skilled and cover it over medium heat. Turn it once until brown for around 4 minutes. Divide the toasted bread over 4 big bowls.

Add in the garlic, flakes of red pepper and stock over to the skillet. Let it simmer.
Get a cup. Break an egg onto the cup and slide the egg over the simmering stock. Do the same thing with the other eggs. Poach the eggs at a slight simmer or up until the egg whites are firm while making sure that each still has a runny yolk. Do this for about 3-4 minutes.

Use a slotted spoon and transfer the eggs to the toasts. Season it with salt. Ladle and place the soup into the prepared bowls and top it with cilantro. Best served with lime wedges.

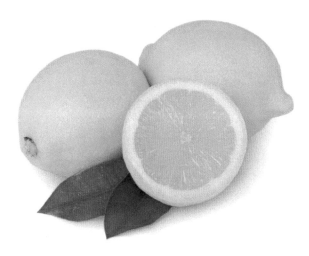

Avgolemono (Lemon Chicken Soup)

Tangy and delightful, you'll love this light but satisfying dish.

Ingredients:
- 8 cups chicken stock
- 1 cup long-grain white rice
- 4 eggs
- Juice of 3 lemons
- Kosher salt and freshly ground black pepper, to taste
- Parsley leaves, for garnish

Instructions:
Prepare a 4 quart saucepan. Boil the stock on high. Lower the heat to medium and then stir in the rice. Cook it while partially covering the saucepan. Occasionally stir it for 20 minutes or until the rice is soft. Whisk in the juice and eggs in a medium bowl until it is frothy. Add in 1 cup of simmering stock and whisk it in until well combined. Transfer it back again to the pot. Cook and stir for 2 minutes more. Add salt and pepper to taste. Top it with parsley.

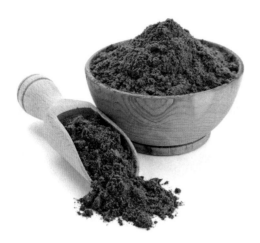

Gazpacho with Smoked Paprika and Jumbo Shrimp

Spicy, smoky and full of flavor, you'll love this seafood delight.

Ingredients:
- 1 28 ounce can or two 14.5-ounce cans diced fire-roasted tomatoes
- 3 cups vegetable broth
- 1 cup V8 or tomato juice
- 2 slices white bread, torn
- 4 small ribs celery from the heart, chopped
- 1 red onion, chopped
- 3 roasted red peppers, chopped
- 1/2 English cucumber, chopped
- 1 clove garlic, grated or finely chopped
- 2 tablespoons sherry vinegar or dry sherry
- Juice of 1 lemon or 1 lime
- 2 tablespoons extra-virgin olive oil
- 2 teaspoons hot pepper sauce
- 2 teaspoons sweet smoked paprika
- Salt and pepper
- Jumbo shrimp, cooked and chilled, for dipping (optional)

Instructions:

Process 1/3 of all the ingredients in a food processor, except the shrimp, salt and pepper, until it is smooth. Transfer it to a pitcher and repeat the remaining ones in 2 other batches. Stir it and add salt and pepper to taste. You can serve it with shrimp, if you are using them.

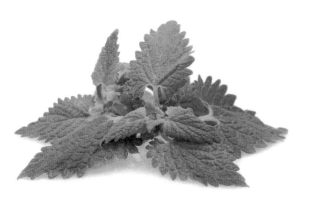

Cucumber Yogurt and Mint Soup

Creamy and delicious, this cool delight is sure to stimulate the senses.

Ingredients:
- 1 English cucumber (peeled, seeded, and finely diced, about 1 3/4 cups)
- 1 tsp salt (divided)
- 1 garlic cloves (small)
- 1/8 tsp freshly ground pepper
- 2 cups low-fat plain yogurt
- 1/4 cup chopped fresh mint (finely)
- extra-virgin olive oil
- 1 whole chives

Instructions:
Mix ½ tsp. of salt and cucumber and set it aside for 15 minutes without draining.

Mince the garlic along with the remaining stir garlic mixture, pepper and ½ teaspoon of salt into the yogurt. Add in the mint. Add in the cucumber and add its liquid to the prepared yogurt mixture while gently stirring. Top it with the chives and olive oil.

Would You Like to Know More

You can learn a lot more about the Mediterranean Diet in my other Best Selling Kindle books. And the best part is that I often will run special promos where I'll offer discounted (usually at $0.99) or free books on Amazon.com.

The best way to get instant notifications for these amazing deals is for you to subscribe to my email list. By signing up not only will you receive info on the latest offer, you'll also get a free copy of this book "*10 Quick & Easy Mediterranean Snacks that take 5 mins or less*". Check out the URL below to learn more.
>>>https://bit.ly/FreeMiniBook<<<

Did You Like The Great Mediterranean Diet Cookbook: Soups & Salads?

Before you go, I'd like to say a big "thank you" for purchasing my book.
You could have picked from dozens of diet books on Amazon, but you took a chance to check out this one.

So again "Thank You" for downloading it and reading the book all the way to the end.

Now I have tiny favor to ask of you. Can you take 1 minute or 2 and give the book a review on Amazon? **Visit this URL to start**: bit.ly/soupssalads

Feedback from readers like you is critical to helping me continue to write the types of books that you want to see. And if you loved the book don't be shy about it.

If you didn't like the book, shoot me an email to let me know why and I'll do whatever it takes to make it right.

Jessica.petras@mavenpublishing.co

Made in the USA
Las Vegas, NV
02 April 2024

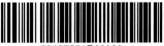

88137351R00026